The Little
Book of
Spiritual
Bliss

To Martha,
My soul sister in bliss

The Little
Book of
Spiritual
Bliss

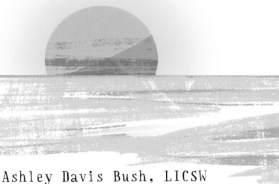

Ashley Davis Bush, LICSW

GAIA

An Hachette UK Company
www.hachette.co.uk

First published in Great Britain
in 2020 by Gaia, an imprint of
Octopus Publishing Group Ltd
Carmelite House
50 Victoria Embankment
London EC4Y 0DZ
www.octopusbooks.co.uk

Distributed in the US by
Hachette Book Group
1290 Avenue of the Americas
4th and 5th Floors
New York, NY 10104

Distributed in Canada by
Canadian Manda Group
664 Annette St.
Toronto, Ontario, Canada M6S 2C8

ISBN 978-1-85675-424-8

A CIP catalogue record for this book
is available from the British Library.

Printed and bound in China

10 9 8 7 6 5 4 3 2 1

Publishing Director: Stephanie Jackson
Senior Editor: Pollyanna Poulter
Art Director: Juliette Norsworthy
Production Manager: Gemma John
Copy Editor: Alison Wormleighton
Proofreader: Jane Birch
Illustrator: Abi Read

Contents

Introduction:
A Spiritual
Anchor

'You are not a drop in the ocean.
You are the entire ocean in a drop.'

RUMI (1207–73), PERSIAN POET AND SUFI MYSTIC

My great-grandfather was a 'cowboy preacher'.
In the early 1900s, he rode from ranch to ranch
on horseback with a Bible in his saddlebag. He
preached, ministered to the sick and baptized
babies. He rode for so many hours, I was told,
that he had to put tobacco juice in his eyes
to stay awake.

He died when I was a child, but I still have a letter that
he wrote to me on the occasion of my birth. He began,
'I would like so very much to see you and instruct you in
some fundamentals in personal conduct but a visit must be
postponed. I will attempt to list a few details here: First, you
and I know that "you came from God, who is your home".
I think others know that, but we are sure.'

He was right – I do know for sure that I came from a
Source beyond myself. I also know for sure that you did
as well, along with every person, creature and plant…
we are all from the same energy, the same light.

But many of us are unaware of this or forget it over time. We get swamped by the details of life, caught up in the whirlwind of chronic stress and 'dis-ease' (an absence of internal harmony, or 'ease'). We live in a world of rampant anxiety and depression, alienation and fear. We fall asleep at the wheel of life, missing the miracles around us. We rarely stop to sit in stillness. We forget where we came from and who we really are.

It doesn't have to be this way. There is a path back to Spirit. Living with Spirit as your anchor is more than just a belief; it's an *experience* of sublime Source in the marrow of your bones. Cultivating a relationship with your spiritual Source becomes a connection that nurtures, sustains and guides you through every aspect of life and even death.

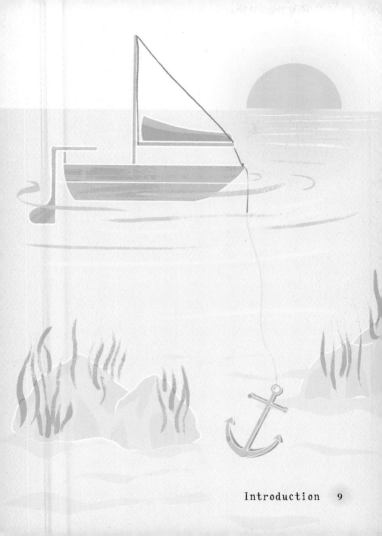

Something More

This book is an invitation to expand your concept of Spirit, going way past the three-letter word 'God' and sensing your way into the benevolent energy that is both beyond you and within you.

God, a name for the unnamable, can have positive or negative associations, depending on your background. Because any one word is limiting and potentially loaded, I'll be using various names for the Mystery of life.

In the end, these words are only fingers pointing at the moon; they are not the moon itself.

Higher Power

Holy Spirit

Mother Nature

Yahweh

Creator

Shiva

Essence

Jehovah

Presence

Allah

Grace

Tao

Krishna

Wise One Lord

Heavenly Being

Goddess

Great Spirit

Transcendent

Divine Mother

Higher Energy

Celestial Light

Consciousness

Universe

Spirit resides in the realm of that which cannot be fully understood with the mind or entirely explained with words. And yet, because it is the very essence of our being, we long for it.

Feeling at one with Spirit creates a deep calm and peacefulness. When you truly know yourself as an extension of Source, you feel beloved and connected to all life on the planet. Your fear recedes because you sense that everything is as it should be, even when it appears otherwise. Life feels easier, full of flow and acceptance rather than resistance and suffering.

Spirituality at Its Core

You have probably already experienced a feeling of connection to Spirit. Think of a moment in your life when you felt completely relaxed, centred and calm...a part of the whole. Perhaps you were in nature – by a lake or walking on a forest path. You may have been alone, with others or with a pet. It might have been a time when you were listening to music or observing majestic beauty. Your heart felt full to overflowing; you were deeply peaceful and calm. This was a spirit-filled experience.

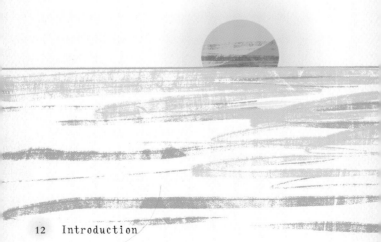

I suspect that when you remember the times that you felt joy, love, gratitude and awe – hearing a child's laughter, watching a sunset, viewing the ocean's ebb and flow – you will know this feeling of connecting to your Source.

The first time I felt connected to Spirit was when I was four years old. I was on a couch with a sleeping puppy on my chest. The warmth, the tenderness, the innocence created for me a sublime sense of peace and connection, of fulfilment.

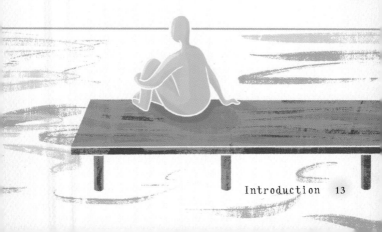

Growing Up with Religion

Spirituality is, of course, quite different from religion. While spirituality is the connection with and expression of Source, religion refers to the human-made, organized rituals, dogmas and traditions that have arisen over time to facilitate that connection.

When I was growing up, I attended a liberal Congregational Church that encouraged ideas such as 'God is love', 'all are welcome' and 'be kind to others'. I was fortunate that my religion aligned with my spirituality, so I felt supported and secure in the religious community. When I look back, I recall experiencing Spirit in the events mostly outside of Sunday services – in the buttered toast served at Friday church dinners and in the music sung with my youth-group choir on Wednesday nights.

Since that time, I have studied and learned from other religious and spiritual traditions, both Western and Eastern: Episcopalianism, Latin American Catholicism, Judaism, Unitarian Universalism, Buddhism, Hinduism, mysticism, shamanism, 12-step spirituality and even Wicca. I have been curious about the multitude of ways that people access Spirit.

There are many stained-glass windows, if you will, between us and the Source of light. While the windows might appear different, each one is illuminated by the same singular light.

Our religious institutions have the power to both deepen and enhance our personal spirituality via inspiring art and architecture, soaring music, sacred rituals, stirring literature and blessed community. Unfortunately, religions have often interfered with the connection to the Divine and even caused terrible damage. Many people feel scarred by their religious upbringing, finding that rather than having experienced sublime connection, they experienced judgement, shame, punishment and fear. As a result, they saw themselves as sinful rather than pure, disappointed and diminished rather than expanded. Perhaps you have experienced this yourself or know someone who has.

Whether you feel weighed down by religious baggage, neutral towards it or uplifted by your religious heritage, this book is your opportunity to find Spirit afresh. It is an invitation to open your heart towards a new sensation of Spirit in every aspect of your life. There is a deep peace – a peace beyond this world – that comes with connecting to Essence every day.

Dropping Anchor

The following six chapters are a compendium of spiritual pause practices that will help you awaken to, connect with and benefit from a spiritual life. The practices are simple and easy and are designed to facilitate your awakening, to encourage you to rethink and recommit to your alignment with Source. The sweet habit of regular pausing, in and of itself, helps you get off the unconscious treadmill of life. And the nature of the practices means that, when they are done regularly, they will create bigger shifts in accessing Spirit.

First, there are practices to help you awaken to your spiritual nature (Chapter 1, page 20) and connect with all things Spirit (Chapter 2, page 34). Then there are practices to help you dwell in wonder (Chapter 3, page 44), love (Chapter 4, page 54) and trust (Chapter 5, page 64). Finally, you will find practices to help you rethink your eternal rest (Chapter 6, page 76), when your time is done on this planet and you transition elsewhere.

Follow these practices in any order, but try to use at least one a day, and preferably two or three. You may find that there is one core practice that you like to use daily, and others that you add or alternate. Trust your intuition to discover what works for you. The main goal is to develop the habit of taking a spiritual pause every day so that you effortlessly and more frequently banish darkness and dwell in light.

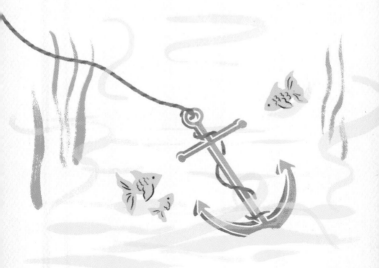

The Benefits of Spiritual Pauses

When you intentionally engage in daily spiritual practices, you…

- Experience a deep sense of inner peace.

- Feel nourished and fulfilled.

- Know there is a purpose to your life.

- Feel connected to and supported by others.

- Reach out to others with compassion.

- Radiate a sense of joy and gratitude.

- Consistently shine light in places of darkness.

- Trust that all will be well (however bleak things might look).

- Know that you're beloved.

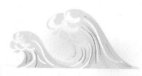

- See vibrant colours instead of grey.

- Have a light to guide you in times of turmoil.

- Know that there is more to life than meets the eye.

- Feel anchored amid the storms of life.

- Become less afraid of death.

Spirit is the ocean and you are a wave among many waves. You are part of the ocean and it is part of you. With the tools in this book, you will drop into the ocean depths so that you can reap the benefits of a life centred in Source. Doing so gives you access to true bliss – joy grounded with inner peace.

Welcome to your life of spiritual bliss.

1. Awaken

'Enlightenment is an accident and practice makes us accident prone.'

ZEN SAYING

When I was 25 years old, I had a spiritual experience. I was on a lunch break from my position as an account assistant for an advertising agency in New York City. I had worked there for only two years but was already feeling jaded, disillusioned, disappointed. Was life really just about selling allergy medicine?

My life seemed like a series of endless, meaningless tasks. I got up every morning, took the subway to work and walked through a sea of people to arrive at my desk housed in a tiny, dark cubicle. My biggest goal was to get promoted from account assistant to account coordinator, a position with a larger, slightly less dark cubicle.

As I sat on a park bench eating my lunch, the sun came out from behind a cloud and illuminated every object and person around me. Everything appeared vibrant, Technicolor, surreal. I looked up, up, up for the source of the light and noticed that everything around me was so *vertical*.

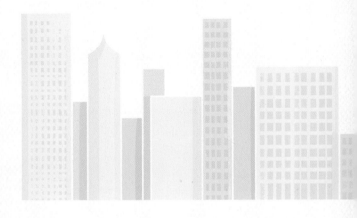

I was surrounded by tall skyscrapers whose windows magnified the light. In that dazzling moment, from the depths of my melancholy, I felt drawn upwards into the light.

In a flash, I was aware that I longed for a more vertical life, a new direction to explore the transcendent. I realized that I had been living along the horizontal plane of life, oriented towards ego and superficiality. But in that moment, I remembered that there was 'Something More' – a spiritual dimension, as vertical as the buildings around me and as full of abundant light.

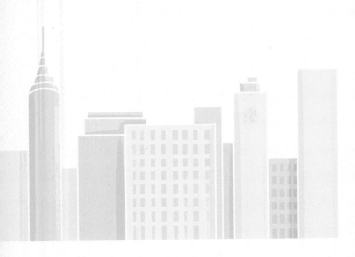

Over the days and weeks that followed, I came to understand that, for me, the vertical dimension meant experiencing the full spectrum of my inner world — from great emotional depths to sublime transcendent heights. It also meant shifting my career to align with my new consciousness.

Although one doesn't have to have a 'vertical' career to live a 'vertical' life, for me it felt right. Within two years, I was a psychotherapist with a spiritual orientation.

Waking up to Spirit means changing your orientation to yourself (seeing yourself as part of something bigger) and also changing your orientation to all beings (seeing everyone else as part of something bigger). When you 'wake up', you see things differently. Previously asleep, you now awaken and perceive everything with fresh eyes.

When you are awake to Spirit, it doesn't mean that you'll never experience pain again, or feel sad, or get sick, or have troubles. You're in a body on this planet, and hard stuff will happen; spirituality doesn't bypass that reality.

However, with a core connection to Spirit, you know that you are not alone — even when you're in trouble. You will be helped, supported, uplifted, watched over, guided, consoled and companioned by Source.

Drawing your strength from a spiritual well means that you can be free — or at least more free — from the tyranny of your ego. When there is less of the false you (ego) and more of the real you (Spirit), then you become less enslaved by the circumstances and challenges of this world.

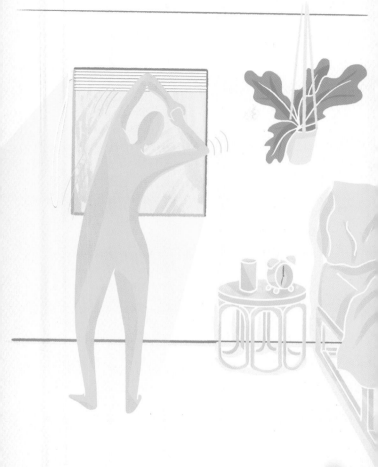

Spiritual Pause Practices

1 Morning Light

Once when I was on retreat in a monastery, I was put in a room they called 'the sick room'. It was connected to the chapel but on the storey above it, with a balcony over the altar. Presumably, it allowed sick monks to lie there while still participating in the monastic services.

Early in the morning, I woke to the sound of monks chanting their morning prayer. *Was I in heaven?* I was mesmerized by the sound of Gregorian chants, and then hymns. Not only did I feel like an angel hovering silently, invisibly, over the small gathering, but I was filled with joy. A euphoric smile affixed itself to me as I absorbed these ancient sounds. It was a singular, transcendent, otherworldly experience that supported me throughout the day.

Of course, most of us do not spend our mornings being serenaded by monks. Still, the energy with which we greet the day matters a great deal. We can jump out of bed, in a rush, swamped by stressful thoughts about what lies ahead – or, worse, immediately check the news or emails. Or we can take an intentional moment to set our course with Spirit.

PAUSE

Before you get out of bed in the
morning, remember the gift of
another day, and put a smile on
your face. Turning the corners
of your mouth up sends a signal
to your brain that all is well.

Next, take a cue from the beautiful
Jewish morning prayer Modeh Ani: 'I give
thanks before You, King living and eternal, for You have
returned within me my soul with compassion; abundant is
Your faithfulness.' Say the words, 'Modeh Ani – I give thanks.'

Yes, you are alive; you are awake; you have another day.
Look around you and see with clear eyes. Notice the beauty
in every detail.

Say 'yes' to life and show up for it. Don't think *What do
I have to do today?* Think *What do I GET to do today?* Have
openness for another day to live, to breathe, to learn, to grow,
to be a light in the world. Send love to your day ahead. *Smile.*

2 Heaven on Earth

Reiki is an ancient energy tool that directs universal life force to promote wellbeing. The Reiki master who lays their hands over you channels life force energy, which activates the chi/qi/*prana* – the spiritual energy that flows within you – as a healing agent. You can stimulate healing energy within yourself by using your own hands as a conduit.

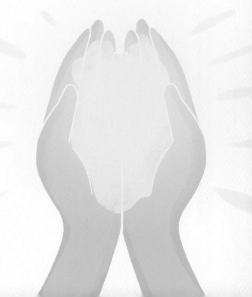

PAUSE

Sit and imagine a warm beam of energy, of pure, benevolent loving goodness, in the form of light. Visualize this force coming from above, down through the crown of your head, down your neck and arms and pooling in your hands. You might feel a warmth or tingling sensation in your hands.

Now cup your palms together and follow these steps:

1. Place your hands over your eyes, covering your forehead and cheeks. Breathe. Rest like this for a few moments.

2. Next, put both palms on top of your head and rest there for a few moments. Breathe.

3. Then put one palm on your forehead and the other palm on the back of your head. Rest. Breathe.

4. Finally, put both hands on either side of your face, touching your ears and cradling your face. Breathe.

Do you feel calm, held, expanded? Can you hold the possibility that you are one with the spaciousness of the universe?

3 Come unto Me

Over 20 years ago, I was on a spiritual retreat in an abbey. A progressive nun led us in a meditation in which we imagined ourselves sitting with Jesus and talking with him. We were to bring our burdens to him and talk to him as a brother.

This particular meditation fell flat for me. I didn't feel inspired. In fact, I felt unnerved and resistant. I didn't want to sit with Jesus. Afterwards, I told the nun that I hadn't been able to connect. She looked at me quizzically, smiled and said, 'How do you feel about the Virgin Mary?'

In truth, I hadn't thought much about the Virgin Mary but I agreed to try the visualization again, this time conversing with Mary. To my surprise, I felt an instant connection. Perhaps it was because we were both women, both mothers – I don't know. But I developed a kinship with Mary after that retreat that has continued to grow through the years.

Our imagination offers us a portal into deep discussions with wise people who are beyond this world. Try the following visualization and notice with whom you connect.

PAUSE

Begin by intentionally settling into the current moment.
As you sit quietly with your eyes closed, notice the sounds
you hear; become aware of your breathing. Now imagine
coming into a beautiful room shimmering with light, where
you meet and converse with a spiritual wisdom figure. You
might imagine a religious figure such as Buddha, Siva, Kuan
Yin, Muhammad, the Pope, a saint or an archangel. Or you
might visualize meeting someone you love who has died, or
a beloved pet; it could even be an ancestor you've never met.
Sit with your wisdom figure and open yourself to their love
– invite a heartfelt experience.

You could choose to sit with them in silence, imagining
their energy, or you might ask them a direct question and see
what kind of guidance you receive. Ask if they have anything
that they would like you to know.

After a time that feels comfortable, thank them for your
experience together. Know that this Being is in your heart
and you in theirs. Know that you are connected. Always.

Breathe; open your eyes; know that you are beloved.

4 Sweet Dreams

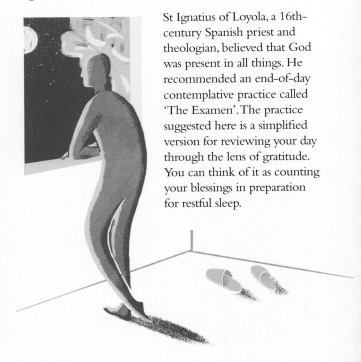

St Ignatius of Loyola, a 16th-century Spanish priest and theologian, believed that God was present in all things. He recommended an end-of-day contemplative practice called 'The Examen'. The practice suggested here is a simplified version for reviewing your day through the lens of gratitude. You can think of it as counting your blessings in preparation for restful sleep.

PAUSE

While you are in bed, drifting off to sleep, try the following:

1. First invite presence by saying, 'Spirit, be with me as I review my day.'

2. Next, recall your day in the spirit of thanksgiving, noticing specific moments of grace, beauty, love, generosity, peace – Spirit-filled moments and experiences that fill you with gratitude.

3. Savour each moment as a gift, and imagine yourself absorbing the feeling of gratitude as you let each snippet sink into your soul.

4. Finally, set your intention for the next day by saying, 'May I be aware of the grace that will be with me tomorrow.' Tomorrow is a new day. You will not wake up exactly the same person as you were the day before. Life is an ever-evolving journey full of hope and possibility.

5. Drift off into a peaceful sleep.

2. Connect

'You have made us for yourself,
O Lord, and our heart is restless,
until it rests in you.'

St Augustine of Hippo (354–430),
early Christian theologian

When I visited Jerusalem, a holy site for three world religions, I was touched by the intense display of deep and abiding commitment to Spirit. I saw Muslim pilgrims with prayer shawls under their arms walking to the Dome of the Rock shrine. I saw Jewish men and women bowing their heads in prayer at the Western Wall. I saw others in line, tearful, as they waited to see the spots where Jesus was crucified and resurrected, both housed within the Church of the Holy Sepulchre.

While it can be awe-inspiring to be present in a place where generations of people have found comfort and inspiration, connecting with Spirit goes beyond buildings, rituals and traditions. As the 13th-century poet and mystic Rumi said, 'I looked in temples, churches and mosques. But I found the Divine within my heart.'

Spirit is like the sun, ever shining. It may be a grey, rainy day but, above the clouds, the sun *is* still shining. Likewise, Spirit is there for you even when you doubt. So why not just turn towards the sun, and connect?

Spiritual Pause Practices

1 Slow and Still

Our society is faster than ever: fast food, fast transportation, high-speed internet…We expect instantaneous communication via texts and emails and nonstop action in our movies and video games. Not only does it seem impossible to slow down and sit in stillness, but it can even feel uncomfortable to imagine slowing down. We wonder, *Won't it be boring to do nothing? Won't I feel restless if I stop?*

Source energy is more easily accessed in slow, quiet moments. And that's why all religious traditions encourage some version of sitting, usually with a calm mental focus (on the breath, a prayer, a word or a chant). By cultivating stillness in this way, the mind settles down, your interior landscape becomes vivid and Spirit can be discerned.

PAUSE

Sit or lie down in a comfortable position. Focus on your breathing, just noticing the in-breath, the out-breath, the space after the in-breath and the space after the out-breath.

Next, repeat the word *maranatha* — an Aramaic word meaning 'come, Lord!' This is a powerful mantra, which you can simply repeat over and over again, syncing it with your breath. Breathe in…'*maran*'. Breathe out…'*atha*'.

Highlighting the presence of the Divine in your meditation reminds you that you don't have to do this world alone. You don't have to deal with your challenges alone, make decisions alone or face your fears alone. You can secure your connection and know that Spirit is with you, around you and working through you, always.

If you prefer a different word to evoke the Divine, choose a word or phrase that rings true. The point is simply to stop the treadmill of your life, to sit and be still, to focus your awareness and to let yourself be saturated with Spirit.

2 Blessing to the Four Directions

This blessing is based on an ancient Native American practice of honouring the earth and the Spirit of the natural world. I first became acquainted with it during a summer solstice ceremony in New Mexico. The Four Directions correspond to the earth elements:

- East/Air: consciousness and insight.

- South/Fire: power, passion, energy.

- West/Water: heart, flow, love.

- North/Earth: solid, abundant, creative.

This is a particularly powerful practice for honouring the morning.

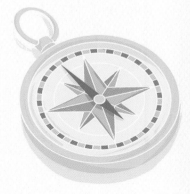

PAUSE

Stand with your hands clasped together. Breathe deeply. Imagine breathing up from the earth, through the souls of your feet, rooting you to Mother Earth. Face each direction in turn, and bow. Silently or out loud, say the following words (or words that resonate with you, if you prefer):

- **Facing East** – 'May I feel the breath of Spirit in the air that I breathe. May I be blessed with higher consciousness, insight and inspiration this day and all days.'

- **Facing South** – 'May I know the power of fire and be filled with energy, joy and strength this day and all days.'

- **Facing West** – 'May I flow like water, free and loving; may I give and receive generously this day and all days.'

- **Facing North** – 'May I be grounded and purposeful and dwell in abundance, this day and all days.'

To finish, lift your arms up to the sky – to the heavens. Now bend your arms down to the ground – the earth. You are linking heaven and earth. And you are at the centre of it all.

3 No One is Alone

You are not alone – not really. You may live by yourself or feel lonely among others, with your ego telling you that you are isolated. However, when you listen for Spirit, you come to know that you are part of the matrix of all life. You are one with all those who cry, who laugh, who survive, who sing, who dance, who celebrate, who get sick, who recover, who age, who mourn and who die. Through Spirit, you are one with all those who lived before you and all those who will live after you. You are a link in the chain of humanity.

St Francis of Assisi, the 13th-century friar and preacher who was known for his love of animals, understood that we are one with the plants, the animals, the sky, the trees, the flowers, the earth. He called to 'Brother Sun and Sister Moon'. You are one with all that is.

Spirit is with you, always. Spirit breathes life into you, accompanies you, watches over you, guides you, comforts you. You are the beloved child of Mother Nature. Even when you believe yourself to be solitary, you are not. Open yourself to the Mystery.

PAUSE

Gaze at a photograph of a person or pet who loves you and whom you love. They might be alive or perhaps they have passed away. Notice how you feel connected, how this loved one is a part of your history, woven into the fabric of you. Say to them, 'We are together in Spirit, always.' Breathe in the feeling state of your connection. Then continue, saying, 'You hold me in your heart as I hold you in mine.'

We are connected to loved ones, to Spirit and to all beings, now and throughout all time. Affirm that, together, you are part of the mysterious whole, that you are one with love.

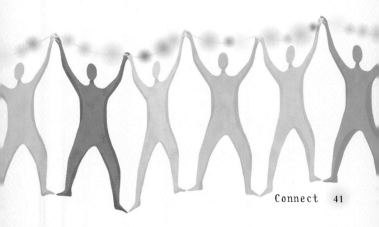

4 Sacred Space

I love to go to monasteries and convents, cathedrals and churches, ashrams and temples, synagogues and mosques. My heart is touched by the explicit devotion, from the grand altars and statues and holy relics to the candles and prayer rugs and flowers. I feel connected to the generations of people who have gathered, uttered prayers, wept tears, engaged in ancient rituals and lifted their voices in word, chant and song.

A space that is intentionally and historically devoted to spiritual practice facilitates a quiet alignment with Source energy. You can make such a space for yourself.

PAUSE

Designate a space in your home where you can create an altar of sacred symbols. Include objects of beauty and special significance, such as incense, candles, crystals, feathers, shells, photos or any items that hold meaning for you. Spend some time – at least five minutes – in your sacred space.

1. Use your senses as a portal to feel the energy. Light a candle, burn some incense and *inhale* the scent. *Gaze* at an icon, statue or image. *Touch* beads, stones or a treasure from nature. *Listen* to Native American flute music, Gregorian chants or the 'Oms' of Buddhist monks. What do you notice or feel that is luminous?

2. Close your eyes and either repeat a mantra or notice your pattern of breathing. Sit in the silence, absorbing the sacred energy of 'Something More'. Can you experience less of your ego and more connection to Spirit? You could 'surrender' a burden to the altar. What you place on the altar gets altered. Write your concern on a slip of paper and place it on the altar. Say, 'Help me release this concern; help me see this differently.' Now surrender the situation and wait for the way to become clear.

3. Wonder

'There are only two ways to live your life. One is as though nothing is a miracle. The other is as though everything is a miracle.'

ALBERT EINSTEIN (1879–1955),
GERMAN-BORN THEORETICAL PHYSICIST

While on vacation by the ocean, I woke at 5am and felt a strong urge to go outside and look at the sky. As I stepped out of the cottage, I was greeted by a sunrise that took my breath away. It began quietly, slowly, with spreading colours of rose and gold that streaked across the sky. From the sea, it seemed, arose the voices of angels, and I felt that I was at the gateway of grace. I was profoundly moved by the magic of it...and yet it was simply another sunrise in August.

Ordinary miracles are happening around you every minute of every day. Babies are born, spring flowers shoot up from the earth, geese honk overhead knowing exactly where to fly – once you open your eyes to see, you'll find that wonder and everyday miracles abound. Practising spiritual pauses creates space for this to happen.

Spiritual Pause Practices

1 Life and Breath

Isn't it a marvel that your body knows to breathe in order to stay alive? Do you know how many breaths you take in a day? In a year? In a lifetime? Isn't it miraculous that your body knows how to do that?

Your breath connects you to Spirit. The Hebrew word *ruach* means both 'breath' and 'spirit'; the Latin root word *spir* means 'to breathe'. Deep breathing activates the body's relaxation response. It calms the central nervous system, both grounding and relaxing your mind, opening you to 'Something More'. A breathing exercise is a perfect way to invite Spirit into your life.

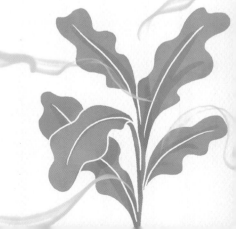

PAUSE

Lift your body upwards by imagining a string at the top of your head pulling you up. Squeeze your shoulder blades slightly together so that your heart centre is open and lifted.

Now try what the Wiccan priestess Phyllis Curott calls 'green breathing' – increasing your sense of reverence and unity with the plants around you.

- Breathe in – imagine breathing in the oxygen from the green plants, the breath of life for us.

- Breathe out – imagine sending carbon dioxide out to the green plants, the breath of life for them.

- Breathe in oxygen, the gift of life from them. Breathe out carbon dioxide, the gift of life for them.

Continue breathing in this way, sharing your carbon dioxide with the plants in your area. Intentionally be part of the continuous circle of life, the circle of breath, the beautiful complete design of nature, of which you are an integral part.

Awareness of unity is only a breath away.

2 Awe-some Pix

When I was a child, I used to love to go to the library and look up old issues of *National Geographic*. The magazine, which has been published continuously since 1888, offered me an intimate window onto our planet. I was mesmerized by the dramatic images of plants, animals, wide vistas, deep sea life and even colourful insects. Without knowing it, I was having a Spirit-filled experience as I flipped through the photographs of beauty and magnificence.

Now, of course, it's as easy as the click of a button to summon an amazing collection of nature images, inspiring both awe and reverence.

Take a moment to use the miracle of modern technology to see the natural wonders of Mother Earth.

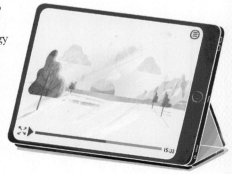

PAUSE

Search on the internet for views of mountains, valleys, national parks, wild animals, wilderness and wildlife gems, 'oceanscapes', different seasons, underwater sea life, rainforests, tropical flowers, rose gardens, birds and insects. Look up majestic sunrises and sunsets, scenes of natural splendour. Investigate the Hubble Telescope pictures of earth, offering a perspective from outer space.

Choose one image and examine it closely. How does it make you feel? Do you notice different things as you let yourself take it in fully? Contemplate how vast and yet how intimate this world is. Absorb the wonder and beauty and give yourself time to be touched by it.

Reflect that you, too, are a part of the sacred design of life on this planet.

3 Eye Candy

Growing up, I had the good fortune to attend a summer camp in New Mexico. For me, the highlight of each trip was to look at the stars at night. I had never seen the Milky Way before – or focused on the vastness of the night sky.

My summer camp was also the home of coelophysid theropod dinosaurs around 200 million years ago. During the days, our eyes were constantly scanning the ground for fossils. In those hot summers, I learned the wondrous value of looking up and looking down, because we never knew what amazing thing we might behold.

You don't need to travel to notice the magical beauty of this world. Look around where you are, right now. This moment holds the key to an experience of wonder and your connection to all that is.

PAUSE

Look up: Looking out of a window if necessary, observe the sky. If it's daytime, how would you describe the colour of the sky? Are there clouds? Do you see the sun? Stop and notice how you *feel* when you look up. If it's night-time, are there stars? Can you see the moon? Do you see any planets? Stop and notice how you *feel* when you look up. There is a vast universe beyond our own planet. How does it feel to be so small and yet an essential part of this amazing design?

Look down: Observe something up close, in magnifying glass detail. If you are outdoors, do you see grass? Flowers? Insects? If indoors, observe an object and drink in each individual facet of it. Is it handmade or machine-made? Notice how, when you take the time to observe something, more details start to capture your attention. Try to see with fresh eyes, as if you are new to this planet and have never come across anything like it before. How does it feel to be so large and yet an essential part of this amazing design?

4 Body Language

Our bodies are miracles of design, with wondrous healing capabilities. Yet most of us grow up with a propensity to criticize, judge and abuse our bodies. We're not thin enough, young enough, pretty enough, strong enough... We might even punish and loathe our bodies.

The following practice invites a shift in awareness towards your body so that you can begin to appreciate the many ways that it serves you in this life. As the poet and mystic Rumi said, 'Why should I be weary when every cell of my body is bursting with life?' Experience the joyful amazement of your body.

PAUSE

Sit for five minutes and do a 'body scan' from the top of your head to the bottom of your feet. Pay attention to your head, neck, torso, arms, hands, heart, stomach, thighs, knees, calves, feet. Where do you notice tension? Breathe into the tense places. Allow your body to relax into the silence.

Each body part works with the other parts to allow you to walk, to heal, to move, to rest. Isn't it amazing that your heart knows how to beat, your body knows how to move blood, digest food, eliminate waste?

Offer up gratitude for the gift of this amazing body, a most useful earth suit while you're on the planet.

4. Love

'What do we live for, if it is not to make life less difficult for each other?'

GEORGE ELIOT (1819–80),
ENGLISH WRITER

One of my earliest teachers about love was Fred Rogers, the beloved host of the American television series *Mister Rogers' Neighborhood*. Rogers uplifted several generations of children with his heartfelt message, 'You are special just the way you are'. He embodied unconditional love and made radical strides in demonstrating that love unites us all.

There is no doubt that we hunger for love. Love is about giving, receiving, sharing, absorbing, forgiving and embracing. Imagine how life would be for you if you knew, deep in your soul, that you were the beloved child of Spirit. Knowing this, you would not only dwell in bliss but also share the love. Imagine life with your heart open, spreading love the way Fred Rogers did.

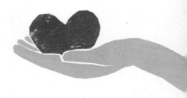

Spiritual Pause Practices

1 Have a Nice Day

I recently made a late-night run to a local shop. As I exited the building, the shop assistant robotically said, 'Have a nice day.' Not looking back, I responded equally robotically, 'You too.' Afterwards, I felt the hollowness of the exchange. Most of us go through life having meaningless interactions, missing the possibility of soul to soul encounters.

Namaste is an ancient Indian greeting which means 'the light in me honours the light in you'. Be open to having a '*namaste* experience' during even the most brief and innocuous of encounters – at the post office, a bank, a café. Any interaction can be light-filled.

PAUSE

When you have even a quick encounter, decide to have a more loving exchange. Mention to the person something nice about the day. Compliment them. Ask a question. If they are wearing a name tag, say their name as you interact.

Imagine sprinkling angel dust in your wake. Wish them loving kindness with sustained eye contact and a genuine smile. Make the moment matter. This person is a soul in a body, just as you are. They are one with Essence just as you are. They also suffer and struggle just as you do. Notice how it feels when you open your heart to another soul.

2 Mirror, Mirror on the Wall

Sometimes it can feel easier to express love
to others than to express it to yourself.
Yet self-love is extremely important.
It is the core of all love that radiates
outwards. As my grandmother
used to say, 'God doesn't make
junk.' You are a child of Spirit.
You are the beloved. The
following practice is about
affirming this truth.

PAUSE

The eyes are often described as the windows to the soul. Look into the mirror, making eye contact with yourself. Say to yourself, 'You are a child of the universe' or 'You are a being of radiant light.' Or use words that work for you to summon a sense of self-love.

If self-love feels challenging, know that many people find it difficult. Happily, though, it can be learned. Try summoning the gift of self-compassion by placing your hand over your heart and repeating the powerful mantra, 'Love is around you; love is within you; you are one with love.' Affirm that you are aligned with a sacred power.

Over time, regular use of this mirror practice will open you to self-compassion, self-acceptance and self-love.

3 Ho'oponopono

This is an ancient Hawaiian practice that calls on the universal powers of remorse, forgiveness, love and gratitude. When the prescribed sentences are spoken as a mantra, and directed towards anyone with whom you struggle, your heart will gradually open. Your relationship will be improved as you surrender resistance and open to compassion. Use the following mantra to shift from negativity to peace, especially when you feel that you have been wronged.

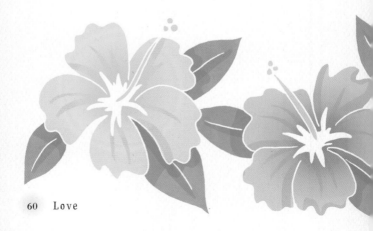

PAUSE

Imagine a person with whom you are having some conflict or who is particularly annoying to you.

Chant the words, 'I'm sorry. Please forgive me. I love you. Thank you.'

Breathe. Repeat the sequence as many times as feels comfortable.

Try doing this every day and notice how you begin to shift and how the relationship, as a result, begins to shift as well.

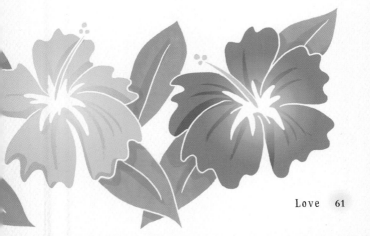

4 Prayers for Peace

A bereaved woman came to see me shortly after the tragic death of her 30-year-old son. We worked together for over a year, in which time her sorrow morphed from searing sharpness to a dull ache. We talked frequently about how living with loss is a part of love and of life. One day she told me that she felt tenderness in her heart and had more empathy. She said, 'Now when I see the grieving people in the news on the other side of the world, I don't just think, *Oh, that's too bad*. I really get it. I do understand their pain in a whole new way – but I still don't know what to do with it.'

She was experiencing deep compassion for other people's distress. Using the following practice, she learned to channel her compassion directly to those who suffer.

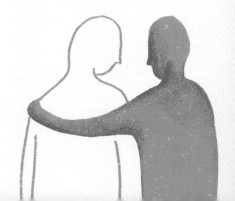

PAUSE

Although you may not feel an instant sense of warmth in your heart, over time, gradually, you will. What you practise grows stronger. Take a moment at the end of this practice to check in with your heart and see if you can detect a softening and a gentle spreading warmth.

1. Sit in a comfortable place and hold your palms upwards.

2. Close your eyes and bring to mind, one at a time, individuals or groups of people who are in need. One by one, picture them in your mind's eye and visualize golden light shining upon them.

3. Hold your hands up and imagine light from your palms radiating out towards them, adding to the cascading light upon them.

4. Say out loud or silently to yourself, 'May you know a deep and abiding peace. May you be surrounded by help and comfort and light. May tender mercies be with you on your journey.'

5. Trust

'All shall be well, and all shall be well,
and all manner of things shall be well.'

JULIAN OF NORWICH (1342–c.1416),
ENGLISH THEOLOGIAN

When you live solely on the horizontal dimension of life, the worldly plane, life can seem overwhelming and even downright terrifying. There are dangers and troubles around every corner. Things that you don't want to change do; and things that you do want to change don't. Life can feel like a cruel game of dodgeball: if you didn't get hit today, you will soon enough.

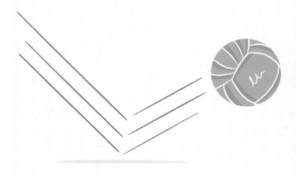

However, when you live in the vertical dimension, on the spiritual plane, you know that things are not always as they seem. You know that challenges hold gifts and that blessings are constantly in disguise.

Some time ago when I was travelling in India, I was on the verge of a painful decision. I was ruminating about it while on a train to Rishikesh when the porter brought along some tea and samosas. Printed in bold letters right on my tea-bag cover was the word 'TRUST'. I blinked twice and thought,

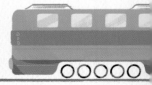

What is happening? Is the universe talking to me? Yes, it felt like a sign for me to TRUST my intuition. I still have that tea-bag cover, and I smile every time I see it.

When you trust Spirit to whisper in your heart, you breathe a sigh of relief. You can turn things over; you can ask for help; you can watch and heed the signs.

Trust takes intention and practice. Use these practices to trust what your heart knows.

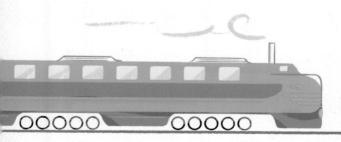

Spiritual Pause Practices

1 Active Acceptance

Acceptance is a process of making peace with the reality of 'what is'. It doesn't mean giving up; it means stopping the resistance to what you cannot change so that you have the energy to open your heart. Acceptance is a form of trusting the universe, even when you don't understand what's happening.

When you choose to go with the flow rather than fight the current, you invite peace. The following practice will assist you in *allowing* and getting out of your own way.

PAUSE

In the spirit of active acceptance, use this practice regularly every time you wash your hands. As the water washes over your fingers, breathe deeply and feel the fluid texture against your skin. Notice the temperature. Now say the following words (either silently or aloud):

'I go with the flow.'

or

'Everything is as it should be.'

or

'May I flow with the river of life without resistance.'

or

'I welcome overflowing abundance into my life.'

2 For Me

Intimate writing orders and distils your experiences, allowing you to reflect in a new way on your life. It activates the observing self, perhaps even your highest self, as you strive to invite perspective.

I have been writing in my journal regularly since I was eight years old. For me, it is a daily habit that soothes my soul. For each of us, journalling has the power to take us into places of discovery where we might not otherwise have ventured.

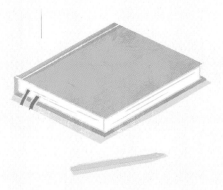

PAUSE

First, reflect on the question, *How might this be happening for me, for my benefit, and not against me?*

Try viewing everything as working for your soul's highest growth, even if circumstances are not as you expected. Ponder how your sprained ankle gives you a chance to rest. Consider how moving house is an opportunity to explore a new life chapter. Invite gratitude towards everything – even things that seem painful and challenging.

Next, journal about your contemplations, whatever thoughts come to mind – even if they are angry, confused or resistant. If you're having trouble seeing how a challenging situation is happening for your highest growth, then write about how you are willing to see things differently, and be open to an eventual shift in perception.

Don't worry about writing in complete sentences – this is just for you. Add the following prompt: 'Why might this be happening *now*, at this particular moment in time, for my soul's growth?' This exercise helps you question your story of yourself as a victim (which is causing your suffering) and illuminates your place as a beloved light connected to Spirit.

3 Candlelight

When I was visiting Kathmandu, I was especially interested in climbing to an ancient religious site called Swayambhunath, known as the Monkey Temple. The complex consists of a domed stupa (which houses relics), various shrines, a monastery, museums, shops and – yes – lots of monkeys.

I was drawn towards a room illuminated by many small flames; I discovered it was the monastery's lamp room, filled with hundreds of yak-butter lamps. As I entered, I heard the chanting bass sound of 'Om' and I literally staggered backwards from the striking beauty.

Candles have been used for centuries to bring light, to cast out darkness, to create atmosphere and to honour special occasions.

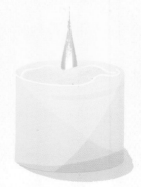

PAUSE

Take a moment to light a candle with intention and reverence.

Mindfully gaze at the centre of the dancing flame. Watching a candle helps to focus your mind and is said to help you attain sublime realization.

As you spend some time with the candle flame, trust the light to dispel your darkness. Trust that there are people who bring light to the planet. Trust that you, too, have a light to share with the world. How is your own light mirrored by the light from the candle?

Blow out the flame and watch the smoke drift into the air. See it as an offering up to the heavens, a thanksgiving for all the many lights on the earth.

4 Make Me an Instrument

In the Christian tradition, the famous Prayer of St Francis begins with the words, 'Lord, make me an instrument of your peace'.

In the Buddhist tradition, the Noble Eightfold Path's route to enlightenment includes 'right livelihood', 'right conduct' and 'right speech'. What you do and what you say directly affects your own and others' suffering in the world.

When you ask Spirit to direct you, you are asking to be of service and trusting that you can make a difference (however big or small). Living in spiritual bliss is a combination of being and doing. Trust that you will be guided to be of service if you open yourself to the possibilities. You have a unique purpose on this planet that Spirit will use in a way that is suited to your gifts. You just need to be open and willing to serve.

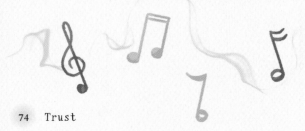

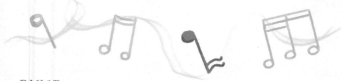

<u>PAUSE</u>

Hold your palms upwards and ask Spirit to work through you, to use you as an instrument of grace on the planet.

- Gesture to the top of your head and ask Spirit to inform your thoughts.

- Gesture to your eyes and ask Spirit to inform your vision.

- Gesture to your lips and ask Spirit to be in your words.

- Gesture to your heart and ask Spirit to open you to love.

- Allow yourself to be an extension of something bigger than yourself. Think of yourself as a flute and allow Source energy to make music through you.

- Notice the areas in your life where you can let Spirit's music play – in your work, at home, with friends and loved ones, with strangers, with animals, with the planet. Mindfully allow yourself to be the instrument.

6. Rest

'To every thing there is a season, and a time to every purpose under the heaven: A time to be born, and a time to die'

ECCLESIASTES 3:1–2

I have spent over 30 years working with grieving individuals. I know that babies die, husbands die, mothers die, brothers die – often without any warning whatsoever. And when it's the right time to leave this earth, you and I will die as well. Guaranteed. This can be terrifying or liberating.

In the 1985 TV movie *Shadowlands* (based on the true story of the author C S Lewis), Lewis recalls how his late wife had told him as she lay dying, 'This is only the land of shadows. Real life hasn't begun yet.' I thought of these words recently with a client who had had a near-death experience. She had died – briefly – on the operating table. Afterwards, she reported hovering above her body and watching the medical team work. She wanted to say to them, 'It's OK. I'm fine.' Then she noticed a light that surrounded her in what she described as 'perfect love'. She felt no pain, no distress, only a sense of profound peace and utter belovedness. It was so lovely, so joyful, that when a 'light being' instructed her to return to her body, she actually felt disappointed.

If you knew that death was an experience of amazing love, incredible peace and supreme happiness, you probably wouldn't fear it so much. And if you could be certain that your loved ones who have died are in a place of profound peace waiting for you to join them, you would rejoice.

Living in spiritual bliss means knowing that when your time comes to die, you will truly rest in peace; all will be well.

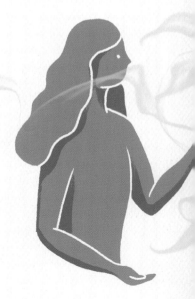

In the meantime, being aware of your mortality – coupled with the certainty that the other side offers peace and grace – can ignite a fierce desire to live more consciously. It's your choice: you can live with awareness that is either clarifying or terrifying.

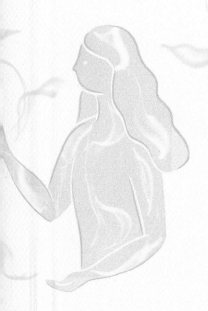

Spiritual Pause Practices

1 Root Lock

The unknown can be frightening, particularly not knowing how and when we will die, let alone what comes afterwards. Yet, it is possible through practice to put our minds and bodies at ease, to ground ourselves in the calm that bridges this world and the next.

The *mula bandha* is an ancient Yogic breathing practice that strengthens your 'roots', leaving you feeling grounded and strong in the face of uncertainty. *Mula* is Sanskrit for 'root of a tree' and *bandha* means 'bond, connect, unite', which is why *mula bandha* translates as 'root lock'.

This variation of the traditional *mula bandha* will help you feel stabilized and calm in the face of any new situation.

PAUSE

1. Sit quietly and take a few deep belly breaths, which are slow and low in your body.

2. Squeeze and contract your pelvic floor muscles (these are at the base of your pelvis where they support your pelvic organs).

3. Lift your pelvic floor muscles vertically, pulling yourself up as if by a string. Draw your navel towards your spine, while continuing to squeeze your pelvic floor. Keep breathing. This motion creates an energetic seal at your root chakra (energy centre) that moves *prana* (life force) into the central channel of your body.

4. Say aloud or think the words, 'I am rooted. I am strong and vertical, like a tree.'

5. Finish with several long out-breaths to expel the air from your lungs.

You may not feel the need to do this every day but be reassured that you can do it anywhere, whenever you feel in need of some calm and stability.

2 Dash

A gravestone in a cemetery typically gives a birth date and death date separated by a dash. Right now, you are living in the dash of your life, sandwiched between birth and death. Are you savouring it? Are you living as you would like? Does it feel like a *dash* – a race to the end?

Poetry is an antidote to the hurriedness of our lives. It uses language to touch the soul and unlock a deeper experience of living.

Poetry – like life – should be read slowly and relished.

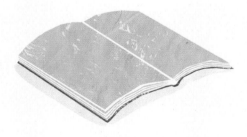

1. Choose a poem from an anthology or online. Select one that reflects on nature, spiritual themes or wisdom traditions.

2. Read it through several times, slowly. Now close your eyes and see how its meaning lands in your heart.

3. Reread the poem. Select one word or phrase that particularly stands out for you. Close your eyes again and sit in silence for a few moments, reflecting on the word or phrase and seeing what feelings it awakens. What does it mean to you? Can you use it for inspiration to live more fully?

4. Invite other poems into your days as a reminder to slow down and appreciate this precious life.

How can facing your mortality inspire you to live more fully now? You don't know how long your life 'dash' will last. What are you waiting to do with your life?

3 The End

'Life is uncertain – death is certain' is a well-known Buddhist saying. In the Buddhist tradition, meditating on awareness of death is said to prepare an individual to meet it as a friend, gracefully.

In the Catholic tradition, a common prayer known as the 'Hail Mary' (or '*Ave Maria*' in Latin) contains the powerful line, 'Holy Mary, Mother of God, Pray for us sinners, now and at the hour of our death.' The reciter of this prayer is reminded of the finality of life, but also consoled by the hope that Mary will intercede on their behalf.

None of us has a choice about *whether* to leave but we do have some choice about *how we face* leaving.

Most of us don't spend much time imagining our deaths, but the following practice asks you to do so deliberately. Do you want to exit this world with fear and resistance? Or do you want to exit with grace and trust?

What if you were to visualize death as a beautiful moment, a moment of blessed transition, graced by peace?

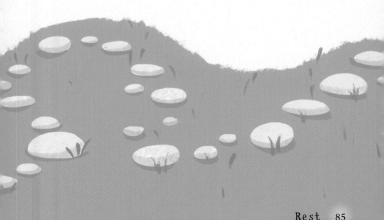

PAUSE

Imagine the moment when you exit this planet, that is, when you die. Allow yourself to be accompanied by one or more wisdom figures – the Buddha, Kuan Yin, Jesus, the Virgin Mary, spirit guides, saints, angels, ancestors, even a dear pet – and visualize them as being present with you and holding you in your dying process. Imagine knowing and trusting that you will not be alone when the final moment occurs. Breathe in the sense of being surrounded by light and peace.

Picture yourself transitioning to the other side, walking across a bridge of light and seeing a dear wisdom figure standing and holding out their arms to you or running towards you. Breathe in the sense of being surrounded by light and peace.

Your moment to join them will come one day, maybe in many years and maybe sooner. You will not be alone. Ask for assistance from Spirit both now, as you contemplate your mortality, and then, at the moment of your inevitable transition. Allow your fears to be soothed with the love and comfort of this communion.

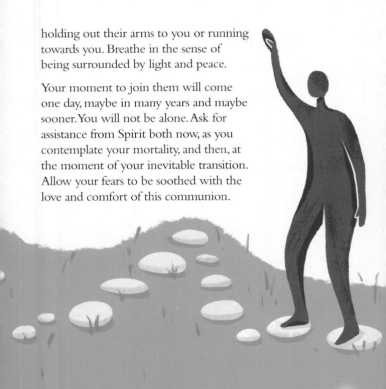

4 Automatic Writing

When a star dies in the universe, its light continues to shine for millions of years. The lights of our dearly departed loved ones shine ever brightly as well.

I have used the following exercise with great effect as I work with bereaved people who are searching for ways to connect with their loved ones.

There is a thin veil between this world and the next. If you open your mind and suspend disbelief, it's possible to lift back the veil.

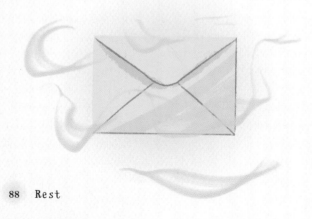

PAUSE

Compose a letter to a deceased loved one, writing it with
your dominant hand. Tell them what you are feeling and
how you are doing since they passed away.

Now dictate a reply letter from your deceased loved one
to you, using your nondominant hand. The reason for using
your nondominant hand is to bypass your inner critic. You
will be forced to concentrate on forming the letters and
therefore less likely to judge the material issuing forth.
What does your loved one want you to know?

While this may seem like a daunting task, try to let the
words flow to paper without thought of composition,
spelling or grammar. Get your mind out of the way and just
let a response come through you. (When psychics are able to
write without consciously doing so, it's known as automatic
writing.) Allow yourself to communicate with a dear one
who is still with you and still part of you. Your vibrant
relationship, based on spirit and love, transcends death.

Conclusion:
A Blessing

'There are two ways of
spreading light: to be the candle
or the mirror that reflects it.'

EDITH WHARTON (1862–1937),
AMERICAN WRITER

Life can seem frightening, lonely and downright pointless when you feel disconnected from your Source. Ultimately, we long to feel a part of 'Something More', to live strongly in the vertical dimension of consciousness.

Even as there are moments of doubt or dark nights of the soul, so also there are moments of illumination. Embrace the possibility within the mystery. Accept the unknowns and uncertainties and fan the spark of hope.

My wish is for you to awaken to Spirit everywhere, viewing life through the vibrant lens of love. I charge you to connect with Spirit every day, to live with an infusion of daily bliss and to know that when your eternal homecoming arrives, all will be well.

Until then, you are here for a reason.

Let Spirit guide and support you.

Further Reading

Adyashanti. *Falling into Grace: Insights on the End of Suffering.* (Colorado: Sounds True, 2013)

Barks, Coleman. *A Year with Rumi: Daily Readings.* (San Francisco: HarperOne, 2006)

Chödrön, Pema. *Always Maintain a Joyful Mind: And Other Lojong Teachings on Awakening Compassion and Fearlessness.* (Boston: Shambhala, 2007)

Curott, Phyllis. *Wicca Made Easy: Awaken the Divine Magic Within You.* (London: Hay House, 2018)

De Waal, Esther. *Lost in Wonder: Rediscovering the Spiritual Art of Attentiveness.* (Norwich: Canterbury Press, 2003)

Fitzpatrick, Jean Grasso. *Something More: Nurturing Your Child's Spiritual Growth.* (Harmondsworth: Penguin Books, 1992)

Frankl, Viktor E. *Man's Search for Meaning: The Classic Tribute to Hope from the Holocaust.* (London: Rider, 2004)

Katie, Byron. *A Thousand Names for Joy: How to Live in Harmony with the Way Things Are.* (London: Rider, 2007)

Lamott, Anne. *Help, Thanks, Wow: The Three Essential Prayers.* (London: Hodder & Stoughton, 2013)

Lief, Judith L. *Making Friends with Death: A Buddhist Guide to Encountering Mortality*. (Boston: Shambhala, 2001)

Linn, Denise. *Kindling the Native Spirit: Sacred Practices for Everyday Life*. (London: Hay House, 2015)

Muller, Wayne. *A Life of Being, Having, and Doing Enough*. (New York: Harmony, 2010)

Rohr, Richard. *Falling Upward: A Spirituality for the Two Halves of Life*. (London: SPCK Publishing, 2012)

Tolle, Eckhart. *The Power of Now: A Guide to Spiritual Enlightenment*. (London: Yellow Kite, 2016)

Weiss, Brian. *Many Lives, Many Masters: The True Story of a Prominent Psychiatrist, his Young Patient, and the Past-Life Therapy that Changed both their Lives*. (London: Piatkus, 1994)

Williamson, Marianne. *A Return to Love: Reflections on the Principles of 'A Course in Miracles'*. (London: Thorsons, 2015)

Acknowledgements

It is with great pleasure that I write about my gratitude for the people who are the wind beneath my wings, who have helped this book take flight, through either direct action, conversation or loving support.

An exuberant thank you goes to Leanne Bryan, Stephanie Jackson, Polly Poulter and the entire talented team at Octopus Publishing. Every project with you is a creative and literary joy! And to John Willig, the best literary agent that an author could ever want, another hearty thanks for your support, your enthusiasm and your guidance.

I bow with thanks to my dear consultation colleagues – Claire Houston, Lesley Zarat and Denise Lamothe – who have not only offered their insights but have patiently participated in the births of multiple books.

I am indebted to the many roots of my spiritual formation: First Community Church, Ghost Ranch, Perkins Chapel, All Souls Church, South Church, Aryaloka, Star Island, the SSJE Monastery, Emery House, Ananda and Adelynrood.

I send my love to the brothers of the Society of St John the Evangelist (SSJE) who have been offering me sanctuary for nearly two decades. I honour my Holy Land Sisters as well as my Spiritual Direction sisters who supported me with their love and prayers.

To my beloved family, I extend my heart in thanksgiving: Peyton and Bill, Sheila and William, Judith and Burton, Rebecca and Taylor, Martha and Stephen, and to my children: Elizabeth, Channing, Setse, Victoria and Inle. I wish for all of you a vertical life of spiritual bliss, always.

And to my lake of calm, my rock and haven, my blessed husband, Daniel. You make every wonderful aspect of my life even better. Spirit moves through you, between us, and keeps our hearts tethered eternally. I am so grateful for your love and support, your attention and abundant generosity. Thank you for your skills in shepherding another book into the world!

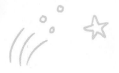

May you live with transcendent bliss. May you feel the brush of angel wings upon you.

May the spiritual pause practices in this book help you on your journey to becoming spiritually attuned and uplifted.

May Source light shine upon you and out from within you... now, always and in all ways.